Asthma Relief Guide: Breath Free, Breath Easy!

Asthma Treatment Programs and Natural Cures

What Is Asthma

Asthma Overview

Asthma is a chronic lung disorder characterized by inflammation of airways, which, in turn disrupt normal breathing patterns. People suffering from asthma have hypersensitive airways, and any irritation in the respiratory system triggers the defense mechanism and blocks these airways, leaving the individual complaining of shortness of breath. Causes of asthma range from simple cold and flu (allergic asthma) to anxiety and stress (non allergic asthma). Asthma attack symptoms include difficulty in breathing, loss of consciousness and chest pain. More importantly, if not treated in time, severe attacks can even lead to death.

The term 'asthma' has been derived from an old Greek word which means 'to pant'. It is basically a chronic condition which affects the air passages when they are stimulated by environmental factors or allergens that act as triggers. There are two particular ways that the air passages respond to asthmatic triggers:

Hyperresponsiveness:

In this, when allergens or any other irritant are inhaled, it results in the smooth muscles in the air passages becoming constricted and getting excessively narrow. Constriction of the air passages when they are exposed to irritants and allergens is a normal reaction that occurs in everybody, however, in people with asthma it results in a special kind of hyper reactive response. In those people who do not have asthma, when an irritant is inhaled, the air passages relax as well as open out in order to expel the irritant from the lungs. However, in those who have asthma, there is no relaxation of the air passages, and instead they become narrow, leading to panting or breathlessness. It is as though there may be a defect in the smooth muscles of those who are afflicted with this respiratory disorder, possibly a lack of some vital chemical, which prevents the relaxation of the muscles.

Inflammation:

Inflammation follows the hyperresponsive stage. When the air passages are subject to allergens or any other environmental triggering factors, the immune system kicks in, delivering immune factors like white blood cells to the area. These cause the air passages to become swollen, fill up with fluid, and produce a sticky, thick kind of mucus. These combine to cause breathlessness, wheezing, the inability to inhale or exhale adequately, and a cough that produces phlegm.

What Causes Asthma

While what exactly causes asthma is still not fully understood, research has shown that it can be triggered by many factors, such as genetics, childhood development as well as growth of the immune system and the lungs, environmental factors, and various types of infections.

Asthma and Genetics:

Scientists and doctors accept the fact that asthma is a hereditary disease. But they have not been able to identify the genes, or gene, that are involved. It is thought that the genes that are associated with asthma are linked to the immune system and the lungs. It is widely known that 'Atopic Diseases', like Asthma, Allergic Rhinitis, and Dermatitis, occur in some form or the other in families.

Asthma and the Immune System:

Research has revealed that the immune system of adults and children who have respiratory problems responds quite differently compared to those without asthma. People who have asthma are generally allergic, and have allergic reactions to factors that cause no problems to others. The immune system of allergic people overreacts when exposed to ordinary substances like cat dander, mold, and pollens. Sometimes, the immune system could even overreact to bacteria and virus, increasing the chances of an asthmatic attack.

Asthma and Childhood:

The initial months as well as years in the life of a child is a vital period during which he/she could become predisposed to developing it. This is due to the abnormalities in the development as well as growth of the lungs. Premature babies are particularly vulnerable to respiratory diseases and infections, since their lungs are not completely developed when they are born. Sometimes, an infection could lead to inflammation, thus injuring the tissues of the lungs.

Asthma and the Environment:

There are several non-immunologic or non-allergic factors in the environment that can trigger the onset of asthma. When a person susceptible to asthma is exposed to these irritants, like secondhand smoke, for an extended period of time, there are higher chances of them developing full-blown asthma. Some of the other such irritants are air pollution, paints, and indoor chemicals.

Research is still continuing to understand how the above factors affect the development of allergies like asthma.

Known Facts About Asthma

Asthma attacks are triggered by exposure to environmental stimulants like cold or warm or moist air, perfume or exertion/emotional stress. In the case of children, it is observed that the common triggers are viral illnesses. The airway narrowing condition causes breathlessness, wheezing and coughing. This airway constriction is eased with the help of bronchodilators. It is common between episodes for the patients to feel well or exhibit mild symptoms.

The symptoms of mild to life-threatening asthma can be controlled with a combination of medication and a change in the immediate environment. Research reveals that in the developed world, this killer is affecting up to one in four urban children! The condition is characterized by chronic respiratory impairment, episodic symptoms triggered by upper respiratory infection, stress, airborne allergens and air pollutants.

An acute exacerbation exhibits clinical hallmarks such as shortness of breath and wheezing and in the late stages of an attack, the air motion may be so impaired that no wheezing may even be heard. If the patient coughs, clear sputum is produced. The signs of an asthmatic episode include prolonged expiration, a rapid heart rate, lung sounds that are audible only through a stethoscope, pulse that is weaker during inhalation and stronger during exhalation and over-inflation of the chest cavity.

During a serious asthma attack, the sternocleidomastoid and scalene muscles of the neck are exerted causing the sufferer to turn blue due to the lack of oxygen. The patient can also suffer the loss of consciousness and just before the loss of consciousness, the patient feels numbness in the limbs and experiences sweaty palms. It is caused by the interaction of genetic and environmental factors. The interaction of these factors influences how severe a person's condition is and the probability of how well the patient is likely to respond to medication.

It is observed that the prevalence of the condition has increased in developed countries with the increase in the use of antibiotics, C-sections and cleaning products. All of these negatively affect exposure to beneficial bacteria and other immune system modulators. There are a number of environmental risk factors associated with asthma. These include traffic pollution, high ozone levels, tobacco smoke and maternal cigarette smoking, viral respiratory infections at an early age, use of antibiotics early in life, cesarean sections and psychological stress.

Many genes are related to the immune system and modulating inflammation. However, research results have not been consistent among all of the population and hence, it is deduced that the genes are not associated with asthma under every condition. Inflamed airways and bronchoconstriction as a result of the inflammatory response cause wheezing. During an asthma episode, the inflamed airways react to environmental triggers and produce excess mucus, which makes it difficult to breathe.

Stimulus to a trigger may include:

- waste from household pests
- pollen and spores
- indoor air pollutants like perfumed products
- soap
- dish washing and laundry detergent
- fabric softener
- paper tissues and towels
- hairspray and gel, cosmetics
- facial sun cream
- air freshener
- oil-based paint
- medication like aspirin and beta blockers
- food allergies
- nitrogen dioxide
- sulfur dioxide

Also, hormonal changes in women associated with the menstrual cycle can worsen the condition though some women experience their asthma improving during pregnancy. Emotional stress can also affect breathing temporarily and so can cold weather and high altitude.

It is recognized that patients who suffer from obstructive sleep apnea and bronchial asthma, often improve when the former is diagnosed and treated. It is cured with the reversibility of the condition that occurs either spontaneously or with treatment. A physician diagnoses the condition on the basis of the patient's clinical history and examination. The measurement of the airway function is possible for adults. Diagnosis in children is based on analysis of the medical history and subsequent improvement. With the proper use of prevention drugs, asthmatics can avoid the complications. However, it is observed that they stop taking preventative medication when they feel fine and this then results in further attacks.

Allergic Asthma

Allergic asthma, is a type of asthma, caused due to the inhalation of certain allergens, such as pollen, dust or dander. The most common type of asthma, it can be also triggered due to inhalation of smoke, fumes or some strong smell. Studies reveal that approximately 90% of children and 50% of adults with asthma have allergies.

Causes of Allergic Asthma

The immunoglobulin E portion of the immune system, in people with allergies, is very sensitive. In such cases, harmless substances, like pollens, are attacked by the immune system, assuming them to be a threat to the health. when encountering an allergen, the human body creates special cells known as IgE antibodies, which trigger the allergic reactions in the body. In this process, chemicals, such as histamin, are released resulting in swelling and inflammation. In case of allergic asthma, the airways in the human body are hypersensitive to allergens. Therefore, the immune system overreacts as soon as these allergens enter the airway. It leads to bronchospasm, a process in which the muscles around the airway are tightened. It also triggers inflammation and thick mucus flooding of the airway. The allergens, in this case, are minute particles which travel to the lungs when a person inhales. Some common allergens are pollen blown by the wind, animal dander, feces of dust mites or cockroaches, animal saliva and mold fragments.

Allergic Asthma Symptoms

The symptoms of this condition can vary from person to person. One person may show different symptoms in two different episodes of asthma. A person suffering from allergic asthma may experience difficulty in breathing, skin rashes, coughing, tightening of the chest, frequent cold, runny nose, sneezing, sore throat, respiratory tract infection and headache. Depression, fatigue, muscle spasms are also common symptoms in this sickness.

Diagnosis for Allergic Asthma

Allergy and asthma tests are recommended to determine the cause of allergic asthma. The most common test involves pricking the skin with little amounts of allergen, and measuring the size of the red bumps that occur 20 minutes later. The blood tests recommended for diagnosis of allergic asthma are radioallergosorbent test (RAST) and the enzyme-linked immunosorbent assay (ELISA).

Allergic Asthma Treatment

It is not possible to completely eliminate allergic asthma, but it can be avoided. Once the cause is determined steps can be taken to reduce exposure to the allergens. Medications meant to treat an allergy can provide relief from its symptoms. Nonsedating antihistamines, like generic Claritin, or decongestant nasal sprays can be used to tackle nasal allergies. If the desired effects are not seen, then nasal steroid sprays and stronger antihistamines, which should be prescribed by the doctor, can be used. If the problem still persists then an immunotherapy (i.e. allergy shots), can be recommended. Inhaled steroids, asthma inhalers, bronchodilators and medicines like Singulair and Accolate pills are prescribed to control asthma. In case of severe asthma attacks, steroids such as Prednisone are administered. Another effective medicament happens to be Xolair, an injectable medicinal drug meant to reduce IgE levels.

Do not use old air conditioners. Pets should be kept outdoors if any individual of the household is allergic to them. Wash blankets, curtains and carpets with hot water once a week. Make sure that the kitchen and bathroom are free from insects like cockroaches or termites. Such simple precautions can ensure your safe health, keeping allergic asthma as well as other diseases at bay.

Cough Variant Asthma

Cough variant asthma is a type of asthma, characterized by chronic and dry or non-productive cough. Unlike asthma, it is usually not accompanied by any symptom, other than the dry and non-productive cough, that can last from 6 to 8 weeks. The typical symptoms of asthma like, wheezing and shortness of breath are usually not observed in the patients who suffering from this condition. The wheezing sound is actually produced when the airways constrict during an asthma attack. But, it may not cause constriction of the airways and hence, it does not necessarily cause wheezing and shortness of breath. However, this type of asthma can cause inflammation and swelling of the airways.

Causes of Cough Variant Asthma

The exact causes are not known properly, though the same allergens associated with asthma such as, dust and pollen can also trigger an attack of chronic cough. Even breathing in cold air can trigger such an attack. Another important factor can be beta blockers, that are used for treating a number of health conditions including, high blood pressure and heart disease. Apart from these, some other important causes are, post nasal drip, sinusitis, acid reflux disease and the habit of smoking. Many times, chronic cough has also been observed to follow an infection of the upper respiratory tract.

Cough Variant Asthma Symptoms

The non-productive or persistent dry cough is the classic and many times, the only symptom. As has been mentioned already, this type of asthma may not present the typical asthma symptoms like, shortness of breath, and the wheezing sound while breathing. But, the dry cough can worsen, particularly during the night and while exercising.

Cough Variant Asthma Diagnosis and Treatment

The diagnosis is a bit difficult. Even X-ray and tests like spirometry or lung function test can show normal results for chronic cough, because of the absence of any blockage of the airways. So, if the results of such test are normal, physicians carry out another test, known as 'positive methacholine inhalation challenge' (MIC) test. In this test, the patient is allowed to inhale methacholine, which causes spasms and narrowing of the airways, in case the patient has asthma. However, even when methacholine inhalation challenge (MIC) test is positive, it cannot be definitely concluded that the person has this condition. The condition is confirmed only when the symptoms responds to usual asthma therapy or treatment.

It is treated with the same medications that are normally used for asthma. Bronchodilators like, albuterol and ipratropium are more commonly used for treating the condition. In addition to bronchodilators, inhaled steroids are also used for treatment. It may take several days for the symptoms to improve or resolve completely. However, occasionally, the cough can worsen in some individuals after using inhaled steroids. Therefore, it is very important to take medications under the guidance of a physician.

Recognizing this asthma is a bit difficult, due to the absence of the usual asthma symptoms. So, if cough lasts for more than 6 to 8 weeks, one should talk to his or her physician, in order to find out and address the underlying causes. Along with the treatment, avoiding the specific allergens like, dust, pollen and even cold air is also essential to reduce the frequency and severity of this condition.

Asthmatic Bronchitis

Bronchitis and asthma are two of the most common respiratory disorders experienced by people. Bronchitis is a disorder of the lungs that occurs when the bronchi, or the air ways in the lungs, get inflamed due to a viral or bacterial infection. Bronchitis can be acute or chronic depending on its causing factor and severity. On the other hand, asthma is also a condition that develops when the airways of the lungs swell or get inflamed. The swelling and inflammation leads to narrowing of the air ways which causes difficulty in breathing. A person suffering from chronic bronchitis and asthma suffers from a condition known as asthmatic bronchitis.

What is Asthmatic Bronchitis

Asthmatic bronchitis is a condition that occurs in people who have been suffering from asthma and contract bronchitis or vice versa. The symptoms of both these conditions are more or less the same, and hence, it is difficult to distinguish between the two conditions. Asthma, bronchitis and asthmatic bronchitis can be triggered off due to several factors like smoking, exposure to air borne pollution like smoke, dust, pollen, mold, etc. As mentioned above, viral or bacterial infection is also one of the major causes of this condition. Asthmatic bronchitis or bronchial asthma is related to Chronic Obstructive Pulmonary Disease (COPD) which occurs when a person suffers from severe and chronic difficulty breathing. The symptoms observed in people suffering from this condition are shortness of breath and difficulty in breathing, cough, chest tightness, wheezing, excess mucus production, etc.

Asthmatic Bronchitis Contagious?

Bronchitis in itself is contagious, but, asthma is not. Asthmatic bronchitis is not a contagious condition. Asthmatic bronchitis, in itself, is not contagious. However, the condition can be contagious if the person suffering from this condition also has a pre-existing respiratory disorder. Therefore, we can say that asthmatic bronchitis can be contagious as well as non contagious, depending on the respiratory disorders that a person suffers from.

As mentioned above, asthmatic bronchitis is not a contagious disorders in itself. However, it should be noted that viral bronchitis can be contagious for 2-4 days. As most of the symptoms of respiratory disorders are more or less similar, it is essential to consult the doctor immediately in case you observe any symptoms. This will help in diagnosing the exact cause and nature of your symptoms.

Treatment for Asthmatic Bronchitis

Although asthmatic bronchitis is not a life-threatening condition, it is essential to take proper medical help in order to prevent the condition from becoming severe. The doctor will advise the person to use bronchodilators to clear the air ways, which will make breathing easier. Secondly, the doctor will also prescribe some corticosteroids and inhalers which will also help treat symptoms like shortness of breath and breathing difficulty. Apart from the treatment methods, there are several preventive measures that need to be followed to prevent activation of the condition. Smoking (active as well as passive) should be avoided completely; one should try to avoid exposure to smoke, dust, or use a face mask; one should vacuum regularly, and stay away from hairy pets.

Lastly, note that nearly all the respiratory disorders can be treated by avoiding smoking and exposure to air pollutions. Secondly, following a balanced diet, and exercising regularly will help in boosting immunity which also helps in keeping infections at bay.

Asthma and Eczema

Did you in your wildest dream ever think that the onset of asthma is linked to eczema. Sounds surprising? That is because both of these medical conditions seem miles apart. Eczema makes the skin inflamed and itchy, while asthma is a breathing problem that is typically marked by inflammation of airways. Although both are a result of exposure to allergens, one cannot ignore the fact that eczema strikes the skin, while asthma affects the lungs. It is hard to believe but the truth is that various studies are convincingly pointing to atopic dermatitis (type of eczema) as the main culprit behind asthma attacks.

The Asthma and Eczema Relationship

Both human and animal studies hint that children catching eczema (atopic dermatitis) may fall prey to asthma in their adulthood. According to animal studies, the section of the skin affected with eczema produces a protein referred as thymic stromal lymphopoietin (TSLP). Unfortunately, TSLP does not remain confined to the superficial skin. It penetrates deeper into the skin and finally enters into the bloodstream. Circulation of blood allows the protein to come in contact with the lungs. When the lungs get exposed to TSLP, it triggers an inflammatory allergic response, leading to asthma. Of course the journey from secretion of the protein TSLP to its accessibility to lungs and the eventual asthmatic response takes years and does not occur within a day or two. Studies suggest that children diagnosed with atopic dermatitis may show asthma symptoms by the time they are nearing 50.

A recent report indicated that every 50 out of 100 children diagnosed with eczema eventually contract asthma. A study that started way back in 1968 and ended in 2004 also hinted that eczema at a very young age could prove to be a getaway for asthma. In this study, health data from over 1000 children (who were 7 years old) was collected. Information about whether they had eczema and hay fever were noted. The same subjects were again evaluated after 34 years to check for any medical conditions. The results that came out were startling. It showed that presently 30% of adult asthma may be due to eczema that was prevalent in childhood.

In yet another animal study, an environment was created so that mice with healthy skin could secrete more TSLP protein in their body. The excess secretion of TSLP eventually caused manifestation of asthma like symptoms in mice. This study again showed that TSLP protein contributes in the development of asthma.

As previously mentioned, animal studies do suggest that TSLP protein has a strong hand in triggering asthma symptoms, but human studies are yet to confirm it. There is no evidence that proves that patients with atopic dermatitis have abnormally high TSLP levels. Doctors are also not sure whether TSLP in humans increases the chance of asthma attacks. The question 'are other proteins in humans also responsible for asthma development' has also not been answered yet. Further studies are needed to clarify these doubts.

Treatment

Is it possible to prevent the itchy eczema from progressing to full-blown asthma? Doctors believe that taking eczema medication at the earliest and stopping the secretion of protein is the key to preventing the onset of asthma later in life. However, medications are yet to be formulated to halt this forward march of eczema that ends with asthma. Nevertheless, early medical intervention to repair the damaged area may stop asthma from occurring. Studies also indicate that people with eczema tend to have a suppressed immune system, which puts them in the risk zone of asthma. Strengthening the immune system by following a healthy diet may benefit in preventing asthma.

Diet can also play a critical role when it comes to managing eczema and asthma. Vegetables like onions, foods rich in vitamin C and E (vegetables and fruits) and seafood (fatty fish) provide anti-inflammatory effect and so their inclusion in the diet can certainly benefit to ease airway inflammation associated with asthma. Also, cook food in healthy oils such as olive oil, instead of corn and sunflower oil. As per the asthma treatment guidelines, the diet should primarily consists of vegetables and fruits and the focus should be less on meat. On the other hand, in case of atopic dermatitis, apart from taking the prescription ointment like anti-itch creams, one should avoid scratching the skin as it may aggravate eczema. Use of harsh skin care products and direct contact with woolen clothes also has to be avoided to manage the skin problem effectively. Eczema is chronic and so may take years to clear away completely. Drinking adequate water and following a healthy diet free from fried food will also help to heal eczema early.

A point to note here is that if a child is diagnosed with eczema (atopic dermatitis), it does not necessarily mean that he is bound to get asthma at some point of time. It only increases the risk of adult asthma to an extent. Further research is awaited that will give a conclusive evidence about the role of TSLP protein in triggering asthma in humans.

Asthma in Babies

We all know about asthma attacks in adults but very few of us are aware of baby asthma. Yes, small babies can develop asthma too. The exact cause is not clearly known. However, much like adult asthma, it is believed that exposure to allergens like dust, smoke, pollen or pet dander are the key causes of asthma in babies and small children. In some babies, it can be triggered by a genetic condition or some physical impairment. As we now know asthma is a respiratory disorder that causes breathing difficulty. It occurs when the air passage gets irritated and inflammation occurs. As a result, the passage becomes narrow and normal breathing gets affected. This causes lack of oxygen in the body. If it continues for a long time, then the body is deprived of oxygen and can lead to damage of vital organs of the body.

Asthma *Symptoms* in Babies

The symptoms of asthma in babies are more or less similar to that of adults. However, as the airway is smaller in babies their intensity is much more severe.

Some of the key identifiable symptoms are given below:

Breathing Difficulty:

As the nasal passage gets constricted, the child struggles hard to maintain normal breathing. It is usually more visible when the baby is crying or doing activities like crawling. The duration of gasping could vary from a few seconds to a few minutes. In a serious asthma attack, it may lead to shallow rapid breathing.

Wheezing:

This is a typical whistling sound that can be heard every time the baby breathes in and breathes out. This clearly suggests that the air passage has narrowed down and only a small amount of air can pass through it.

Cough:

A chronic cough which could be dry or wet. They may cough occasionally throughout the day but it may worsen during the night. Laughing or crawling may also trigger it. This cough may be accompanied by other allergy symptoms such as sneezing, watery eyes and nasal discharge.

Tightness in Chest:

As there is less amount of air available in the lungs, the baby tries to put extra efforts into breathing in more air. This often results in chest tightness.

Allergic Rashes:

When tiny, red skin rashes appear on various parts of their body like the cheeks, forehead and scalp, along with other asthma symptoms then it clearly suggests that he or she was exposed to some kind of allergens which is causing the attack.

Spasms:

Infantile spasm is quite commonly associated with baby asthma. It can be described as contraction of one or more muscle groups of the body for a short period of time. If it is a severe spasm that lasts for several minutes, then the baby should be rushed to the hospital.

There are some serious symptoms that require emergency medical intervention.

They are as follows:

- Rapid breathing
- Retraction or drawing in of the stomach towards the ribs
- Widening of the nostrils
- Bluish discoloration of lips and nails
- Paleness in face

Treatment

The moment you suspect that your little child has developed asthma, you should consult your pediatrician for further treatment. They diagnose baby asthma by studying the symptoms, medical history and family history of the child. The main aim of the treatment is to help the baby deal with the asthma attack. Doctors prescribe suitable medicines, which when administered to the baby at the onset of the symptoms, can stop the attack. These medicines act quickly and provide relief from the spasms inside the air passage. It enables the baby to breathe easily. There is a device called metered-dose inhaler (or MDI) which is being used for administering the medicines directly into the airway. It consists of a small aerosol can which has to be inserted into a long tube with a small mask called spacer. The mask is placed on the baby's face and the medicine is sprayed into the spacer which the baby inhales while breathing through the mask.

If your baby tends to get asthma attacks frequently, you must take steps to prevent any such attacks in future. Identify the allergen or the condition that causes the attack. Some babies get it when they are infected by a common cold. Others may get it on exposure to dust or tobacco smoke. Once it is identified, try to make every effort to ensure that your baby is not exposed to that particular allergen.

Asthma in Toddlers

Causes and Symptoms

As mentioned earlier, this condition might run in the family. Environmental pollution, frequent exposure to cigarette smoke, changes in the weather, infections such as fever and flu, allergies, etc., are usually the triggers. As per the surveys conducted by various health institutions, the risk of asthma increases, if the mother continues to smoke during pregnancy.

In case of some toddlers, a wheezing cough can be a prominent indicator. The affected child may show reluctance in playing games or activities which would require him/her to move a lot. In most cases, affected children seem to dislike physical activities that are strenuous such as running and playing games that involve running.

This might be accompanied by other symptoms such as:

- Difficulty in breathing
- Flared nostrils
- Inability to feed well due to breathing distress and muscle retraction
- Rapid breathing during sleep

If your child complains of labored breathing, wheezing, coughing spells, and tightness in the chest, you should bring it to the notice of a pediatrician immediately. These symptoms should not be ignored.

Treatment

Since children who are under the age of 5 years cannot undergo pulmonary function tests, doctors usually conduct a physical exam, and also analyze the child's medical history. The treatment usually involves the use of inhaled corticosteroids or combination inhalers. The main objective is to avoid the potential triggers of an attack, but if a child suffers from an attack, the use of short-acting bronchodilators is suggested. These medicines help in widening the airways and facilitate proper breathing. Parents must ensure that the child has a quick-relief inhaler with him/her at all times. Medicines must be administered as per the guidelines given by the pediatrician.

In many cases, it has been observed that asthma resolves as these children grow up. In other cases, one must always be prepared in the event of an attack.

Asthma Attack in Young Children

Asthma is known to be more common in young children than in babies. Almost 9 million children in the United States alone suffer from asthma. A number of factors contribute to children being more prone to developing this disorder, most commonly at the age of 5 and some even at a younger age. Asthma in children can be quite a discomfort and it is essential that parents know how to prevent the same in children. The symptoms of asthma in children may be a bit more severe than in adults and emergency medical treatment may be required to get these under control. Here are the causes, symptoms and treatment options of asthma attack in children.

Causes

The causes of asthma attacks in children are similar to the causes of asthma attacks in babies and adults. Asthma attacks are a result of, or triggered, by an exposure to allergens like smoke, pollution, dust and pollens, a change in weather conditions, respiratory infections and emotional disturbance. Mostly, allergens is what triggers the attack. Children are more prone to developing chronic asthma due to their underdeveloped respiratory system and small airways. They can develop asthma in case of allergies being present or a family history of asthma and boys are more prone to being asthmatic than girls.

Symptoms

The most common symptoms are also very similiar to those found in babies and adults. They include severe wheezing when breathing in or breathing out, troubled or rapid breathing, chest tightness and coughing. These symptoms tend to worsen during the night and breathing may get increasingly difficult. Asthma in children often goes undiagnosed as these symptoms are considered to be associated with other respiratory disorders as well. Medical assistance may be required if the breathing condition of the child does not improve and signs like the lips and nails turning blue are noticed. In children below the age of 5, the most common symptom of asthma is an upper respiratory infection like a common cold. If asthma in children goes untreated for a while, it may get severe and cause many problems for the child during his or her adulthood. In most children, asthma attacks lessen in frequency or can even disappear completely during their teenage, but returns after that and could be difficult to treat at this point.

Treatment

Treatment can be administered in a number of ways. The most common asthma treatment option is the use of inhalers for asthma that help broaden the airways and breathe easily, thus reducing the symptoms. In case of a severe asthma attack, the child should be put on a nebulizer until he or she finds it easy to breathe. Corticosteroids may also be helpful in relieving symptoms during an attack. Drugs like theophylline and aminophylline, Beta 2 agonists and anticholinergics are safe and can be administered to asthmatic children.

Tips for Prevention

If you are aware of the fact that your child is asthmatic and wondering how to deal with asthma attacks, you should take the following preventive measures to avoid triggering an asthma attack in your child.

- Determine what triggers an attack in your child and take adequate steps to prevent the child from being exposed to these triggers.

- Take immediate action and administer medication as soon as you notice any of the symptoms.

- Treat respiratory infection and minor colds and cough immediately so that an asthma attack can be prevented.

- Educate the child about the allergens and irritants that can trigger an asthma attack in him or her.

- Keep your home, especially the child's bedroom and play area clean and dust free by vacuuming it on a daily basis.

- Monitor the child's lung function by using a *peak flow* meter. You can also determine if the child is at a risk of an asthma attack with the help of the readings of this device.

An asthma attack can also prove fatal if it is not treated on time or can have long-term consequences on the health of the child. Try to prevent these attacks as much as possible with the help of medication and regular monitoring.

Asthma Symptoms in Adults

Although, childhood asthma is the most common form of asthma, adult asthma is also not unheard of. There are several causes of adult asthma but like the in the others, allergens are considered to be the primary cause. When the air is inhaled through the nose, it is warmed, filtered and humidified. This air then passes through the trachea and further gets divided into right bronchus and left bronchus. Each of these, then leads to small tubules which further branch into thousands of very small tubules. Inflammation usually occurs in the large and small tubules. When any irritant enters these inflamed air passages, they get constricted, cutting off the air supply to lungs. Let us now review and understand the symptoms of asthma in adults, in detail.

What Causes Adult Asthma

When a person above 20 years of age is diagnosed with asthma, he is said to be suffering from adult asthma. There are various reasons why it may surface in your adult life. You may have had asthma in childhood but never had any symptoms. Though, it is possible that mild asthma symptoms may have been mistaken for some other illness. During adult life, you may suddenly become sensitized to certain allergens, which trigger the symptoms of asthma. Usually, people who experience hormonal changes or just recovered from a prolonged illness are more susceptible to exhibiting adult onset asthma symptoms. Women who are pregnant or just delivered a baby may show adult asthma symptoms. Similarly, women nearing menopause or those who have been on estrogen treatment for more than 10 years have an equal possibility of developing asthma. People who recovered from a bout of flu or viral infection are also at the risk of developing asthma. People with pet allergies especially cat allergies may develop asthma. Certain occupational hazards may also trigger bronchial asthma.

Adult Asthma Symptoms

The severity of asthma symptoms in adults may vary greatly. Some people may only suffer a mild breathing problem, while others may experience severe symptoms that warrant a doctor's intervention. It is uncommon for the symptoms to appear abruptly, as they usually have a tendency to develop within hours or days of exposure to the asthma trigger. Given below are some symptoms of asthma in adults.

- Most of the asthma attacks are characterized with wheezing while breathing air out. As wheezing and rapid breathing becomes more severe all the respiratory muscles become visibly active.

- Shortness of breath is another common symptom experienced by adult asthma patients. The severity of these symptoms does not necessarily imply the damage to bronchial tubes. In fact, many people are not even aware that they are experiencing shortness of breath. Such people are at a greater risk of developing a life-threatening condition. Mostly women in the age group of 50 to 60 fall in this category.

- Coughing is also experienced by many asthma patients and find it particularly distressing. Incessant, nonproductive coughing can interfere with the sleeping pattern of the person.

- A sudden, unexplained chest tightness may be an early indicator of an approaching severe asthma attack. About three quarters of patients also report chest pain prior to an asthma attack

- Another symptom includes stiffening of neck muscles which makes it impossible for the person to talk.

- Asthma attack is also characterized by sweating and rapid heart rate.

Adult asthma is diagnosed on the basis of medical history of the patient. A breathing test is also performed in which the amount of air inhaled and exhaled is measured with a device called a *spirometer*. Certain other tests are also effective in measuring the performance of the air passages. Lung X-rays may also be helpful in diagnosing adult asthma. Bronchial asthma symptoms and treatment are often in accordance with these tests results.

Adult asthma symptoms may occur anywhere, anytime. Hence, if you have a known allergy to an irritant, take due precautions after getting exposed to that irritant.

Guidelines for Asthma Treatment

Formulate a Treatment Plan

As soon as a diagnosis of asthma is made, the first and foremost thing that needs to be done is the formulation of a treatment plan. This will be specifically given by your doctor. The treatment for the condition will be formulated depending on the underlying cause that is triggering the asthma attack. However, more often than not, environmental pollution and certain allergies are the most common culprits, though psychological stress has also been implicated in certain cases. Depending on the severity of the condition and the underlying trigger, it is classified as acute or chronic, after which the treatment plan is formulated.

For acute attack cases of asthma, short acting beta agonists, such as albuterol is usually given in the form of metered dose inhalers. Anticholinergic medications can also help those cases that exhibit severe symptoms. For chronic cases, more often than not, with the help of certain maintenance and prevention measures, the frequency of attacks can be brought down to minimum. That brings us to the second and equally important part - prevention and patient education.

Patient Education & Prevention

As they say, prevention is better than cure. This is the main reason why patient education and prevention of asthma episodes go hand in hand. As each case is unique in nature, the person first needs to identify the trigger factor that leads to these attacks. Thus, the person must at all times, avoid coming in contact with cigarette smoke, pet fur or any kind of allergen that may be the cause of his asthma attacks.

In the long run, asthma treatment plan will stress on slowly bringing down the frequency of attacks to a bare minimum. For this, the best option available is to make use of glucocorticoids. This is a type of steroid that helps prevent occurrence and exacerbation of asthma attacks. Yet another option is to include the use of long acting beta adrenergic agonists, which manage to stay effective for around twelve hours. These beta adrenergic agonists, however, need to be used in conjunction with steroids so as to prevent taking any risks of attacks.

The drug safety office of the FDA suggests that this class of drugs should be removed from the medications list given when there is an asthma attack in children. Other drugs that are only used in cases where mild symptoms are seen and where the frequency of attacks is minimal include leukotriene antagonists and mast cell stabilizers. Eating healthy and ensuring that the immunity of the person is not compromised at any stage is equally important, as these may be the factors which are co-responsible for an asthma attack.

The prognosis of asthma is largely dependent on the severity and frequency of attacks, and how well they are treated and controlled. The earlier this condition is diagnosed, the better is the prognosis. Although many people may feel that this is a highly enfeebling condition, it is not actually the case. Provided an early and effective treatment plan is made, one can always live a normal and healthy life, with minimal occurrences of asthma episodes.

Asthma can be quite frightening and certain steps need to be taken to avoid complications. The treatment is simple but its timing is very important. One must identify what triggers one's asthma such as pollen, dust, smoke etc. Hence, it is best to stay away from areas which can trigger the attack. Also some people are more prone to attacks during particular season, this can be avoided by taking extra care.

Treatment Without Inhaler

To treat asthma without inhalers, first thing one must do is to identify the symptoms. The sooner one identifies the symptoms, the better. The next thing to do is to distance yourself from the asthma trigger. Sit in a well ventilated place and do not panic. Try and breathe slowly, if you find it difficult to breathe, calm yourself to bring the heart rate down. Take a paper bag or something similar and try breathing with that.

If you have an anti-allergic medicine or an asthma medication with you, then take the medication. Once the breathing gets relatively easier, try to get an inhaler. Remember to always carry it with you, no matter what. The best way to treat asthma is to not panic yourself or make the patient panic, especially during an attack in a child.

Emergency Treatment

In case of an emergency treatment during an asthma attack, do not make the person lie down. Do not crowd around the person, try to make him sit, so that it is easier for him to breathe. The next thing is to make the person use his inhaler. For an adult, 6 to 7 puffs will suffice, whereas for a child, 4 to 5 puffs are enough. If there are any asthma triggering factors around the person, such as dust or even a pet, distance the person from them for the time being. Once the breathing has returned to normal, medication should be administered immediately.

Home Treatment

This is a quick run through for home asthma treatment. Later on we will go over these in more detail.

There are many home remedies for asthma. If one detects the onset of an attack, then drinking something hot like black coffee or soup can really help the person. Some people greatly benefit by increasing vitamin C, vitamin B12 and vitamin B6 intake in their diet which help to prevent the attack. Reducing the intake of salt also helps in the same way.

Hot honey and ginger also help clear the passage ways, and since the throat is clear, breathing is much easier. Of the many home remedies is inhaling the fumes of juniper oil dissolved in hot water for some instant relief. Mixture of mustard oil and camphor, if rubbed on the back also helps during an attack. Caffeine helps in clearing the airways, so drinking coffee is a good idea.

Inhalers for Asthma

An asthma inhaler is a hand-held device which provides asthma medication directly into the airways. The medications can be taken orally and intravenously, but with the inhaler the medication goes straight into the lungs and quickly relieves the patient from the symptoms with minimum side effects.

There are varieties of inhalers available and they mainly fall into two categories:

Metered Dose Inhalers (MDIs)

Metered dose inhalers utilize a chemical propellant to propel an evaluated dose of medication out of the inhaler. They comprise a mouthpiece, a pressurized canister having medication and a metering valve which dispenses the right dose of medication. The medicine is released either by inhaling or squeezing the canister. Some inhalers have counters to know how many doses are remaining. If there is no counter, the patient needs to keep a track of the number of doses used, in order to know when the inhaler would be out of medication. The chemical propellant commonly used in metered dose inhalers are chlorofluorocarbon (CFC). But since it damages the ozone layer, other propellants like hydrofluoroalkane (HFA) are now been used. The dose of medicine released by HFA inhalers is more soft, warm and reaches directly to the lungs.

Dry Powder Inhalers (DPIs)

Dry powder inhalers do not have a gas propellant to propel the drug out of a canister. Each dose contains a small amount of drug in a powder form, which the patient has to suck in. The patient has to breathe in very hard to get the powder into his lungs. Most adults and older children find it easy to operate, but young children may find it difficult to breathe in so hard and suck in the powder. These inhalers may be difficult to use especially during an asthma attack, as during such times it is hard to catch a deep breath anyway. On the other hand, some find them easier as compared to the metered dose inhalers, as the hand-lung coordination is not needed. The different types of dry powdered inhalers include a powder disk inhaler, a dry powder tube inhaler and a single-dose dry powder disk inhaler. Spacers are not required to be used with these inhalers.

Inhalers with Spacers

A spacer is a tube which is attached to the inhaler and holds the medicine until the patient doesn't breathe in completely. It gives more time to inhale slowly and decreases the amount of medication that deposits on the back of the patient's throat and tongue. It makes the use of the inhaler simpler and helps in depositing the medicine into the lungs more efficiently. In this, the hand-breath coordination is not important and deep and fast breathing is not required. This type of inhaler requires regular cleansing with soap and water.

Asthma inhalers have transformed the treatment of asthma and other lung diseases. They are the most effective way of providing life-saving medication to the patients. Although there are hardly any side effects, it is always advisable to consult a doctor before using any type of inhaler.

Asthma Inhalers Over the Counter

Over the counter asthma inhalers are considered to be quick relief medication that help to reduce the symptoms within a few minutes. However, these inhalers are highly effective for those people who suffer from mild asthma, i.e., patients who do not take regular asthma medications and/or experience symptoms less than twice a week in a day. These asthma inhalers without prescription primarily include epinephrine, also known as adrenalin, a medicine that relaxes the muscles located in the airways and helps the person breath easily. In addition to epinephrine, at times an expectorant which helps in opening the airways by loosening the mucous is also included in some over the counter asthma medications.

Though these inhalers provide instant relief from asthma symptoms like wheezing, their effect last only for a few hours and if not used properly they may cause some side effects. Research shows that occasional use of these over the counter asthma inhalers is safe and effective but gross or improper use of these products can result in adverse effects, including death. Basically these inhalers stimulate the heart, and cause increased heart rate and blood pressure. Hence, for people who are already suffering from heart diseases, these inhalers can be hazardous, and so such patients should use these inhalers carefully and should avoid using them frequently.

Apart from these, another treatment option is taking tablets containing ephedrine, a drug that relaxes and dilates the bronchial passageways and improves the passages of air into the lungs. The tablet is directly taken into the mouth and is absorbed through the stomach. The main advantage of these tablets over the inhalers is that the onset of action is more gradual and last for a longer duration of time. Also the medication has comparatively less side effects as compared to asthma inhalers.

Though over-the-counter inhalers for asthma are easily available, and extremely useful and quick in overcoming asthma symptoms, it is strongly recommended to consult your doctor before using them in order to avoid overuse or misuse of these epinephrine-based inhalers as this may cause adverse reactions in patients. Also despite providing instant relief, these inhalers are best suited to patients suffering from mild asthma, i.e., who use them occasionally, as their long term or frequent use can keep the patient from seeking proper medical care from their doctor which indeed will worsen their asthma.

Beta Blockers and Asthma

Beta blockers are a group of medications that are used to treat various forms of illnesses and ailments including blood pressure, heart problems, glaucoma, hypertension and migraines. They are also known as beta-adrenergic blocking agents because they tend to block the effects of the adrenaline hormone in the body. By blocking the adrenaline effects, the beta blockers can help the heart muscles relax and improve the flow of blood circulation. Because of their ability to relax the muscles, they prove to be extremely beneficial for treating angina, heart attack, anxiety, hyperthyroidism, and few other conditions that call for 'relaxation'. Some of the most common beta blockers are - Atenolol, Acebutolol, Nebivolol, and Metoprolol. But why do beta blockers cause a problem for people suffering from underlying bronchial asthma? Can asthmatic patients not use these medications to treat their illnesses?

Beta Blockers for Asthma Patients

Our body contains three different types of beta-receptors known as β1, β2, and β3 receptors. The β1 receptors are located in the heart and the kidneys, followed by the β2 receptors which are located in the liver, lungs, skeletal muscles, uterus, gastrointestinal tract, and the vascular smooth muscle. The β3 receptors are found in the fat cells of the body. Now, there are two types of beta blockers that are available, the non-selective beta blockers and the selective beta blockers. As the name signifies, the non-selective beta blockers can block multiple types of beta receptors in the body. On the other hand, the selective beta blockers are designed to block only selective types of beta receptors in the body. Some sources state that cardio selective beta blockers are actually safe for asthmatic patients to consume. On the other hand, experts suggest that though the selective beta blockers are more safe than non-selective beta blockers, there is still a risk for them to cause severe health problems. Therefore, be it selective beta blockers or non-selective ones, people with asthma should avoid this medication at all times. Apart from not being appropriate for asthma patients, these medications are also not advised by healthcare specialists for people suffering from diabetes. This is because these drugs tend to relax the heart muscles, thereby blocking the signs of low blood sugar levels or hypoglycemia in a diabetic patient. Fluctuations in the blood sugar levels of a diabetic patient should be carefully monitored, and beta blockers may pose a problem in doing so.

When a person is suffering from a condition like asthma, other signs and symptoms like anxiety and sleeplessness can occur. Both these conditions result from the shortness of breath and discomfort that occurs in asthma patients during attacks. In this condition, sleeping pills and tranquilizers are something that the patient may ask for, however, make sure that you don't go for them at all without medical supervision! As far as beta blockers are concerned, some people also use certain short-acting beta blockers for sleep related problems which should again be avoided. So, make sure that you completely avoid beta blockers if you have asthma. It is always best to consult with your doctor for alternate medications and remedies.

Beta blockers, as it is should be taken with a lot of care and caution as there are several side effects that are associated with beta blockers and their usage. While some people experience problems like fatigue, headaches, diarrhea, dizziness, constipation, and cold hands and feet; there are some people who do not experience any problems at all. In fact, some people who do not have asthma but consume these medications also experience shortness of breath and sleeping problems. Which is why, beta blockers are also known to flare up asthma in patients with underlying bronchial asthma. So, always make sure that you consult a trusted healthcare specialist before you go ahead with using beta blockers for treatment.

Bronchial Thermoplasty

Bronchial asthma is an inflammatory disease that affects one's airways and causes the sufferer to experience a variety of discomforting symptoms such as coughing, wheezing, shortness of breath and tightness of chest. While mild asthma might be manageable, in severe cases, it could give rise to a life-threatening situation. When one suffers from an asthma attack, the airways get inflamed to such an extent, that these might get constricted and the person might experience severe breathing problems due to an insufficient supply of oxygen to the lungs. Though asthma can be treated with the help of inhalers or bronchodilators, sometimes these may not provide relief.

Studies have been ongoing for developing an effective treatment option for chronic bronchial asthma. Bronchial thermoplasty is one such treatment that is currently being used on those who haven't benefited from drugs. Wondering how does this non-drug procedure help in treating asthma? Here's some information about the effectiveness of this procedure for the treatment of severe asthma.

Procedure

Asthma treatment generally involves the use of inhalers that deliver small doses of corticosteroids so as to reduce the inflammation in the airways. If the use of inhaled steroids or other asthma medications doesn't seem to help, doctors might recommend this procedure. This is a minimally-invasive procedure that is performed under mild anesthesia. It is performed in three outpatient procedure visits. A device called a bronchoscope is passed through the nose and throat. Once the bronchoscope passes through the airway passages and is properly positioned in the lungs, a catheter is inserted. The catheter's tip is inflated so that it comes in contact with the sides of the airway wall. The catheter acts as the vehicle for the delivery of the ablating agent, which in this case is the radio frequency energy. The smooth muscle walls of the airways are then heated to a temperature of 149 degrees Fahrenheit. This aim of this procedure is to minimize the contraction of the airway smooth muscle. It is the constriction and contraction of this muscle that causes the airways to close. When that happens, the lungs don't receive sufficient amount of air and one suffers from breathing problems. Thinning down the smooth muscles of the airways limits the ability of the airways to constrict and that provides relief from the discomforting asthma symptoms.

Benefits and Side Effects

Since this bronchoscopic procedure is a relatively newer treatment, clinical studies are still going on to determine the effectiveness of this non-drug procedure for asthma control. Though this treatment does help in reducing the intensity of an asthma attack, it is not a complete cure. You will still experience the symptoms if asthma triggers are around. However, you will notice a considerable change in the intensity of asthma attacks. Some studies indicate that patients who had undergone this procedure paid fewer visits to the emergency room. Though the studies have revealed that this treatment considerably reduced the severity of the symptoms and did improve the quality of life of the patients, the long-term effects of this treatment are yet to be found out.

The ideal candidates of this treatment are people suffering from severe asthma. It is recommended only if drug therapy has been found to be ineffective. This bronchial asthma treatment is not meant for those who haven't completed 18 years of age. As is the case with any medical procedure, this bronchoscopic procedure can also cause certain side effects. For instance, delivering radio frequency can result in certain side effects. It might irritate the airways or cause a lung infection. Some people might experience side effects on account of administration of anesthesia. Though life-threatening side effects have not been seen, but long-term side effects are still not known. If you are suffering from chronic bronchial asthma, you can consult a pulmonologist to find out more about this procedure. Each treatment will cost you around $1,500. Since most people require a minimum of three sessions, you might end up paying anywhere between $4,500 to $5,000.

Bronchial thermoplasty has given hopes to those suffering from severe bronchial asthma. Though the long-term effects of this bronchoscopic procedure will be known only after elaborate studies are conducted, some of the clinic studies reveal that it has improved the quality of life for chronic asthma sufferers.

Bronchodilator Treatment

Bronchodilators are the medicines which are mainly used to treat asthma. The airway passages in the respiratory tract which transfer air into the lungs are called 'bronchi'. These passages further divide into minute tubes called 'bronchioles'. Bronchodilators help widen the bronchi and bronchioles, increasing airflow to the lungs. The use of a bronchodilator results in decreased resistance in the airway passages, and thus facilitates easy and unobstructed respiration.

Bronchodilator Types and Uses

Beta-agonists, anticholinergics, and theophylline, are the three main types of bronchodilators. They are ingested in the form of tablets or liquids; or are injected or inhaled. As these medicines help open the bronchial tubes, air can flow easily through lungs. Most people prefer to inhale beta-agonists and anticholinergics. Short acting bronchodilators provide quick relief to the patients of asthma. A person who often suffers from asthma attacks can use them in asthma nebulizers. Long-acting bronchodilators help manage and control asthma symptoms for extended hours. Some of them are known for their instant effect, while some may take about 30 - 45 minutes to begin working. Their effect may last for more than 12 hours. As air moves freely within the bronchi and bronchioles, mucus gets cleared from the lungs. It becomes easy to cough out the mucus, once it starts moving freely. Some bronchodilators (anticholinergics) are used to treat COPD (disorder caused by excessive smoking) in emergency rooms. Some bronchodilators like theophylline exhibit mild anti-inflammatory properties and help lower inflammation of the lungs. Side effects of bronchodilators are usually noticed after consumption of too much of medication.

Bronchodilator Medication Side Effects

Although bronchodilators are used to treat respiratory problems, their overuse can result in life-threatening side effects. Albuterol inhaler side effects include skin rash, hives, itching sensation, blurred vision, diarrhea, stomach ache, indigestion, nausea, headache, constipation, rapid or irregular heart rate, chest pain, tightness of the chest, etc. Side effects of theophylline are also similar. Excessive use of theophylline may lead to muscle pain, stomach ache, muscle cramps, fatigue and nervousness. It may result in hyperactivity as well. A dry throat is one of the most common side effects of atrovent. Eye contact with the medication can lead to burning sensation in the eyes, and it may cause vision problems too, for a short period of time.

Some of the most common side effects of bronchodilators include irritation in the throat, dizziness, light-headedness, heartburn, breathing difficulty, loss of appetite, altered taste sensation, restlessness, anxiety, nervousness, trembling, and sweating. Sometimes, such side effects are noticed initially when the person starts using bronchodilators. But as the body gets adjusted to these medicines, the side effects subside and disappear eventually. Long-acting β2-agonists (for example, Salmeterol and Formoterol) are usually taken twice a day with an anti-inflammatory medication (inhaled or oral). The bronchodilators may increase the risk of death if they are taken regularly without a steroid. Some bronchodilators interfere with routine medications, leading to various side effects.

Asthma patients need to avoid both normal smoke and cigarette smoking. Otherwise, the medications will be of no use. Orally taken bronchodilators exhibit more side effects than asthma inhalers because they contain higher doses. Oral bronchodilators need to be present in the bloodstream in order to reach the lungs. Thus, the chances are higher that they lead to certain side effects; as the same blood is transferred to each and every organ. But bronchodilators obtained from asthma inhalers are transferred directly into the airways in the lungs, and therefore they exhibit fewer side effects.

Bronchodilator side effects may vary according to the type of bronchodilator used and the overall health of the person. Side effects of these medicines may vary depending upon how much medication is taken or inhaled. Excessive use of short-acting bronchodilators, in any form, indicates chronic uncontrolled asthma. Overuse of these medicines indicate that the person needs more aggressive treatment. If you need to use bronchodilators more frequently, you should consult your physician immediately.

Prednisone for Asthma Treatment

Drug therapy is one of the most common forms of treatment for various ailments that affect mankind. When doctors prescribe drugs, their main aim is to alleviate the symptoms of the disease and prevent the disease from progressing any further. In fact, some of the pharmacological agents that help in restoring the natural bodily processes are versions of the chemicals that are synthesized within the body. Prednisone is one such synthetic glucocorticoid that produces the corticosteroid-like effect after it is ingested. The mechanism of action is similar to that of the corticosteroid hormones that are synthesized by the body. Since this drug basically helps in regulating the inflammatory response of the body, it is used for the treatment of inflammatory conditions.

What is Prednisone Used For?

Prednisone is one of the most commonly prescribed synthetic glucocorticoid drugs. It suppresses the inflammatory response that occurs in response to injury or pathogenic infections, which is why it is also referred to as an immunosuppressant. It is basically an inactive derivative, which gets processed into an active metabolite called prednisolone. The chain of events that either occur as a part of inflammatory response or occur when the immune system becomes overactive, can be stopped with the help of this drug. Since it is an anti-inflammatory drug, it is used for the treatment of conditions such as asthma, allergies, ulcerative colitis, Crohn's disease, endocrine disorders and rheumatoid arthritis. Since it acts as an immune suppressant, it may also be prescribed for the treatment of autoimmune conditions. Its use is recommended after an organ transplant as well. This is to prevent the body from rejecting the organ, and preventing the inflammation that may occur if the immune system recognizes the implanted organ as a foreign body.

Prednisone for the Treatment of Asthma

Asthma is an inflammatory disorder of the airways which is characterized by shortness of breath, coughing and wheezing. Inhalation of environmental irritants such as smoke, dust, chemicals, pollen or anything that one may be allergic to, may trigger an attack. The air that we inhale, passes through the trachea, and is then taken into the right and left lung through right and left bronchial tubes. An asthma attack occurs whenever one inhales anything that irritates the airways and causes them to get inflamed. As a result of inflammation, the airways tighten and become constricted. Excessive production of phlegm may also occur as a result of inflammation. This gives rise to breathing problems. Those who are asthmatic may also experience symptoms such as coughing, wheezing and tightness of chest during such episodes. Under such circumstances, inhaled corticosteroids, oral corticosteroids, bronchodilators or nebulizer medications are prescribed in order to dilate the airways and bring down the inflammation. Prednisone is usually recommended for those who suffer from severe symptoms.

Is It Safe to Use Prednisone for Asthma?

As mentioned earlier, this drug is recommended in case of an acute asthma exacerbation. An attack can be life-threatening if the airways become constricted and cause respiratory distress. It is definitely one of the most potent, synthetic corticosteroid that can help in suppressing the inflammation, however, long term use of this drug must be avoided. While some patients may experience untoward effects due to an allergic reaction, long term use can even have an adverse effect on one's immune system. Since it acts like an immunosuppressant, prolonged use of this drug can make one vulnerable to infections. While a steroid burst, wherein high doses are given for a few days will certainly prove beneficial, using it for long periods of time certainly poses many health risks. Doctors are well aware of the problems related to long term use of prednisone for the treatment of this respiratory condition which is why they exercise caution while recommending this drug. While the prolonged use of this drug can affect a child's growth and may even affect the body's ability to produce natural corticosteroids, fluid retention, thinning of bones, easy bruising, abnormal weight gain, fatigue, muscle weakness, diabetes mellitus and cataract are some of the side effects that may occur due to prolonged use. One must also take the steroid as per the recommended dosage and take it until the time that has been suggested by the doctor. One could even become highly dependent on this drug, and may develop withdrawal symptoms if one stops using the drug suddenly. Thus, doctors reduce the dosage over a period of time, before the long term treatment is stopped.

Though asthma is a common condition that affects adults as well as children, it can be controlled with the help of drug therapy and self-care measures. Avoidance of the triggers is the best way of preventing an attack. Usually, steroids are prescribed when the use of other drugs are not giving the desired results. If doctors do prescribe a steroid such as prednisone, they prescribe short burst of this oral steroid. The main aim of short burst therapy is to reduce inflammation, while avoidance of triggers will help to reduce the frequency or recurrence of asthma attacks in future.

Magnesium Sulfate for Asthma

Asthma, that is typically marked by trouble breathing, is a condition in which the air passages (tubes) that transport inhaled air into the lungs get swollen. To be more specific, swelling strikes the inner walls of airways. The swollen airways restrict free flow of air, thereby making it difficult to breathe properly. One of the best ways to manage this life long medical problem involves use of medications like corticosteroids and bronchodilators that are inhaled to get relief from shortness of breath. However, when this first line of treatment doesn't work, especially when it is an acute asthma attack or refractory asthma, doctors go for magnesium sulfate.

Acute asthma is not easy to manage, especially when the person is being treated at home. An acute asthma attack is sudden and the symptoms progress rapidly to life-threatening consequences. Studies show that magnesium sulfate is found to be useful in the management of acute asthma. So, in order to prevent complications in acute asthma, treatment with this chemical compound is definitely safe and when taken in the right dosage, does not produce any major side effects. The person may experience mild to moderate physical discomfort at the site of administration.

Treatment

Severe cases of asthma may not respond to conventional treatment. In such circumstances, using magnesium sulfate has proved beneficial to control acute asthma. As we all know, in asthma the muscles surrounding the airways contract abnormally. This condition is referred as muscle spasms that prevents air from moving freely in and out of the lungs.

Studies show that magnesium sulfate given intravenously, promotes relaxation of muscles. Besides reducing muscle contraction, the chemical compound also helps to decrease the swelling of the inside walls of the airways. This positive result is observed with intravenous administration of magnesium sulfate alone and also when it is given in conjunction with bronchodilators.

Severe asthma attack can be life-threatening if treatment is delayed. A worsening asthma attack is a medical emergency and desperate measures need to be taken to improve breathing. So, if bronchodilators or corticosteroid medicines fail to provide any relief, administering magnesium sulfate is advised.

A point to note here is that magnesium sulfate is an alternative to bronchodilators but long-term use of magnesium sulfate is discouraged. Also, in a study, it was observed that magnesium sulfate is not very effective in controlling non severe cases of asthma. Hence, inhaling bronchodilators or corticosteroids is always a better option when it comes to managing mild to moderate asthma. There is no need to use magnesium sulfate when asthma can be controlled with standard asthma attack treatment. Magnesium sulfate comes into picture only when the conventional treatment seems to be ineffective in relieving asthma symptoms.

Dosage

Many ask, in what dose magnesium sulfate should be given intravenously so as to restore normal breathing pattern. Approximately 50 ml of saline water will contain 40-100 mg/kg of magnesium sulfate infusion. This dose should be given intravenously for approximately 20-30 minutes. A 45 mg/kg dose often works to treat refractory asthma in children. However, this dose might be given again as required to control severe asthma exacerbations. Adult dosage may vary from 1.2-2g/kg IV magnesium sulfate and is administered for around 20 minutes. On the whole, administering intravenous magnesium sulfate infusion at the desired rate as instructed by the doctor can promote better lung function.

Apart from asthma treatment, magnesium sulfate has quite a few other medicinal purposes. For instance, it is useful to treat pregnancy complications like eclampsia. Oral or intravenous administration of magnesium sulfate is also used to alleviate symptoms of magnesium deficiency. Application of solution containing magnesium sulfate also helps in improving skin problems like acne.

However, the uses of magnesium sulfate are not just restricted to medicinal purposes. It has a wide range of industrial application that vary from preparation of warm salt water in flotation therapy to production of gun powder.

Caffeine as an Asthma Treatment

The relation of caffeine and asthma is one of the hotly debated topics in medical science. While most original studies have concluded that the effect of caffeine is not beneficial for managing asthma symptoms, some newer studies have come to light which report otherwise. The reason some scientists have proposed that the use of caffeine may help people with this respiratory condition, is the former holding some properties that are similar to that of theophylline (a long-acting bronchodilator, that relaxes and dilates the bronchial passageway thus, making it easier to breathe). Theophylline is a medicine that is prescribed for controlling and managing spasms of the airways; a common symptom in people with asthma and COPD (Chronic Obstructive Pulmonary Disease). Also certain studies have reported that caffeine has anti-inflammatory properties, which is yet another point that may establish its benefits for asthma.

Effects of Caffeine On Asthma

As mentioned above, many recent studies have been able to exhibit the effect of caffeine on asthmatics as a bronchodilator. One of such studies was conducted on about 8 adult patients, who were diagnosed with asthma symptoms. The patients either received placebo or caffeine, and as long as 8 hours after the drink, various tests were conducted on the patients. And when the results came in, it showed caffeine showed significant improvements in managing the symptoms, as compared to the placebo effect. But what has to be considered here is, despite having so many effective drugs against asthma, why are scientists so much focused on something such as caffeine. There are two main reasons behind this. The first being that, if caffeine is actually helpful in relieving asthma flare-ups, then it could be a better choice than medications. The second, and probably, a more important reason lies in the fact that, consumption of caffeine may affect the nature of tests or diagnosis conducted to determine how bad someone's asthma actually is in the present situation. What happens normally is, caffeine when taken in small amounts, is known to stimulate lung function thereby improving it for up to four hours. So this means that, if a person consumes the same before undergoing a test for lung function (which is important in determining the stage of his asthma), he would show better results. So if in reality the patient's condition requires a stronger asthma medication, he might be prescribed with a weaker drug, given his improved lung function in the test. So needless to say, this might create significant problems in managing the condition.

The association of caffeine with asthma is an ongoing study, so that medical experts can help people understand if the former product really helps in improving asthma symptoms, and if they should or should avoid taking caffeine before going for tests to determine the function of their lungs. So it is always better to consult his/her healthcare provider before attempting to manage this condition with caffeine.

Fish Oil for Asthma Treatment

Asthma is one of the leading diseases taking over the American health today, costing it as much as $13 billion every year. Almost 5000 deaths are caused annually by asthma alone in United States. Moreover, it does not have a cure. Its symptoms can only be diminished with a proper diet with special supplements and alternative therapies.

About Fish Oil

Fish oil is the richest source of omega-3 and omega-6 fatty acids that have anti-inflammatory properties and are essential for a healthy diet. Its main constituents are docosahexaenoic acid (DHA) and eicosapentaenoic acid (EPA) that are used by the body to repair and produce new cells. Did you know? The occurrence of asthma in Eskimos is remarkably lower as compared to the statistics around the world. This can be attributed to their diet which is rich in omega-3 and omega-6 derived from cold water fish.

Certain oily fish that are beneficial for asthma treatment are Atlantic salmon, Hoki, sardines, mackerel, mullet, rainbow trout and orange rough. They contain more than 2% fat and should be consumed at least 4 times a week.

Benefits of Fish Oil for Asthma

According to a research, supplementing an asthma patient's diet with fish oil reduces the symptoms of lung inflammation. The average daily dosage of fish oil for the treatment, recommended for significant improvement in breathing, is 3.3 grams everyday. The advised quantity not only improves the condition of asthma patients but also reduces the risk of the disease when consumed daily during childhood. Daily intake can prevent severe asthma attacks by reducing the constriction of the bronchi-oles and puts you to ease. You will see results in 2 months.

It is proven and documented by scientific research that you cannot substitute this oil with omega-3 and omega-6 supplements to reap the benefits. The body has to convert them to long chain acids, that is DHA and EPA acids, to use them.

Therefore, this oil is preferred over flax-seed oil. It's not just the fatty acids that play a role in preventing or reducing asthma, but there are other components in the fish oil that are unknown yet but are major asthma fighters. However, if you are allergic to fish or do not like to eat it, you can opt for capsules.

In fact, in Hyderabad, India, there is an annual festival in the month of June wherein a particular Goud family hands over live fish dipped in a paste of special herbs to thousands of asthma patients. The special 'medication' is said to improve asthma among people who are prescribed a strict diet regime for the next 45 days. The family proclaims it to be an exotic and powerful recipe passed down over generations as an asthma cure and refuses to share it with pharmaceutical companies. This oil is especially beneficial for children and women in their late pregnancies.

Avoid eating fried fish though. Broiled or grilled fish is a good choice for your health because frying it can take away its nutrients. Fish oil for treatment of asthma is completely natural and so it can be taken with your regular asthma medication with no side-effects. Please note, the use of fish oil is not recommended for people ailing with depression, bipolar, HIV/AIDS and diabetes as it causes blood thinning. Excessive intake may also cause vomiting and nausea.

How to Treat Asthma During Pregnancy

Asthma is a chronic disorder of the respiratory system where periodic inflammation occurs in the air passage and normal airflow into the body gets affected. It is triggered due to irritation of the lining of the air passage caused by allergens, irritants, infections, cold weather conditions, hormonal changes and so on. An asthma attack is identified with symptoms like breathing difficulty, wheezing, chest tightness, cough, etc. Asthma attacks during pregnancy is fairly common. Those women who have a medical history of asthma tend to get the attacks more frequently during pregnancy. On the other hand, some women develop asthma during pregnancy.

Many women try to avoid asthma treatment during pregnancy as they feel that medicines can cause harm to their unborn baby. It is true that taking asthma medicines may not be good for the baby but an uncontrolled asthma attack during pregnancy is even worse. It decreases the amount of oxygen supply to the mother and the fetus. This can lead to serious complications like high blood pressure in the pregnant mother, pre-eclampsia, low birth weight of the infant, premature baby birth, etc.

For treatment during pregnancy, you have to involve both your pulmonologist and the obstetrician. Do not stop taking medicines on your own when you come to know about your pregnancy. Rather, you must inform your obstetrician about the medicines that you are taking. When you inform your pulmonologist that you are pregnant, then he or she may change the dosage of the medicine or give you new medicines.

The most popular medicine used for treating asthma during pregnancy is steroid inhalers. It opens up the air passage and alleviates symptoms. It may be accompanied by oral steroid medicines or injections. The dosage of these medicines depends on the frequency of the asthma attack and severity of the symptoms. Do not worry as your doctor will select suitable medicines for you that have minimum side effects on you and your baby.

If asthma is triggered due to exposure to allergens, then doctors prescribe antihistamines for controlling the allergy symptoms. A nasal congestion due to upper respiratory tract infection is often treated with oral decongestants. Those who are prone to flu attack may be advised to take flu shots to prevent aggravation of the problem. Regular intake of medicines is not enough, you also have to visit your pulmonologist to monitor the lung function from time to time. Your obstetrician will also recommend frequent ultrasounds to check fetal growth.

How to Stop an Asthma Attack

Although there is no foolproof way to keep an asthma attack from occurring, avoiding factors that trigger the attack, and taking medications as prescribed by the doctor reduce the risk to a great extent.

The first preventive measure is following the treatment plan that has been recommended to you by your doctor. Asthma can be managed by two types of medications; the long-term ones, and the short-term ones. The short-term medicines are used to control an attack. It is the long-term medications that are used to prevent an asthma attack. In most cases, these medications need to be taken on a daily basis. It is important to understand that the condition is a lifelong one, and thus requires constant monitoring and management.

The next important step to be followed is identifying triggers, and avoiding them. Although experts are still dubious about the specific causes of this chronic condition, they are well aware of the factors that may trigger an attack. Substances such as pollen, dander, dust, mold, cold air, air pollutants, smokes from tobacco, incense, candles, fires, and fireworks, and food allergens are known to trigger an asthma attack in most people. Some people may experience an attack, after they get exposed to infections such as common cold, due to medications, and diseases such as gastroesophageal reflux disease (GERD). Strong emotions and stress, may cause the same in some people. Even indulging in physical activities may induce an attack. Cockroaches, indoor mold growths, and dust mites are some other triggers. For instance, if you experience an attack usually after exercising, then it is better to stop any such activity, and stay away from it. Try going for something less intense such as walking or jogging. Also, getting a flu shot every year would do good to you, as infections such as this may worsen asthma symptoms. Likewise, getting allergy shots may also be a helpful preventive measure.

In some people, some symptoms may indicate an impending asthma attack. So getting familiar with all the warning signs and symptoms, would provide a great deal of help in reducing the risks. These signs could be a slight coughing, wheezing or difficulty in breathing. Pain in the chest could also be a sign. It is best if you can predict an attack even before these signs occur. And this can be done by monitoring your breathing rate. For this, you can avail a home peak flow meter.

A slight reduction in the frequency of attacks does not warrant you to stop the medications. Irrespective of any improvements or not in the condition, it is a must to complete the course of medication as prescribed.

The only and the best way to deal with chronic conditions such as asthma is to prevent it, with constant effort and monitoring. Following the above steps in the right way, may not always guarantee to prevent an attack, but they would definitely cut down the risks significantly. Next I will give you a step-by-step instructions on how to tackle an attack before it gets detrimental.

Step #1: Calm Down

While this may seem very repetitive and practically impossible to do in the midst of an asthma attack, it is the first step that you need to take towards stopping an ongoing attack. Most often what happens is when a person feels the onset of an attack, he instantly panics. When he panics, it automatically increases the heart rate, which further contributes to the severity of the attack. So, when you're in the thick of one, first calm down and then follow the other instructions given below.

Step #2: Distance the Trigger

Once you have calmed down, you will be able to think clearly. Now, slowly look around and identify what has triggered off the attack. You will be well aware of the triggers that you get affected by. It could be dust, pollen, pollution, food, allergens, a particular scent, smoking, or even excess physical movement. If it's dust, pollen or such triggers, then immediately create a distance between yourself and the trigger. Go out of the room which contains the trigger and into an area that has ample supply of fresh air. If it's due to exercise or any other physical movement that has caused the attack, then stop the movement and rest your body to bring down the blood rate.

Step #3: Breathing Exercises

Once you have settled down away from the trigger of your attack, you can indulge in some simple breathing exercises that will help your breathing get back to normal and in turn, make the attack subside. A couple of these exercises have been given below.

1) Sit down and hold your nose with your hand. Shut your mouth and hold your breath. Now, slowly shake your head in an up to down motion. Continue this until you feel suffocated. Then, slowly release your nose and slowly take in breath. If you cannot breathe through your nose, then let go of your nose, purse your lips and take in a little breath from the corner of the mouth. When you feel better, begin breathing slowly through your nose. Repeat this exercise after about a minute or two until your breathing reaches its regular pace.
2) This second exercise involves sniffing in and out. You need to sit in an upright position with your hands on your knees. Bend forward a little and inhale 4 short sniffs. After you're done inhaling, you need to straighten up a

bit and exhale one long breath. Then again bend a little and repeat the procedure twice before resting for about 10 seconds. Continue this exercise for about 10 minutes when you experience an attack, and you'll feel better.

Step #4: Get Assistance

If any of the steps given above fail and you feel like your symptoms are getting aggravated even after using an inhaler, check your peak flow meter to see what your respiratory condition is. If it reads below the required reading, rush to your doctor immediately. Waiting for an asthma attack to subside on its own can only be stretched for some time. You are the best judge of its severity. So, don't take any chances prolonging the period of discomfort.

The best way to stop an asthma attack is undoubtedly preventing one in the first place. So, stay away from all the possible triggers, take your medication regularly, keep your inhaler at hand and your emergency numbers with you all the time. Avoid too much physical and mental stress and live a healthy life.

Pre-Treating an Asthma Attack at Home

Along with the medicinal treatment, you have to take a few remedial measures at home to control asthma symptoms. A few helpful tips in this regard are as follows:

- Strictly avoid tobacco smoke exposure. Those pregnant women who are smokers should quit the habit immediately. Smoking can lead to a severe asthma attack.

- Make sure that your home and office environment where you spend maximum time is free from environmental irritants like dirt, dust, pollen, mold, etc.

- Do not go outdoors in cold weather conditions. If you have to go, make sure you cover up your mouth and nose properly with a scarf.

- Mix some rock salt with mustard oil to prepare a thick paste. Massage this paste gently on your chest daily. This reduces the chances of an asthma attack to a great extent.

- Garlic can provide relief from asthma. Boil 8-10 garlic cloves in a glass of milk for 10 minutes. Let it cool down and then drink it. It should be taken daily for best results.

Home Remedies for Asthma Attacks

These remedies generally aim at providing relief from asthma attack by using readily available food items, herbs and some precautionary measures to tackle the breathlessness associated with asthma. Given below are some simple remedies which resort to readily available ingredients to relieve you of the complications associated with this respiratory ailment.

- One of the most popular asthma attack cures is drinking a cup of strong black coffee. This is one of the natural cures for asthma which will keep the situation under control until the patient is provided with medical help.

- During an asthma attack, adding juniper oil to hot water and inhaling its fumes can help in providing much-needed relief for asthmatics.

- Other than juniper oil, people suffering from asthma can also add caraway seeds to boiling water and inhale the fumes as a home remedy for asthma attack.

- Studies have revealed that vitamin B6 and B12 are helpful in reducing inflammation of lungs, therefore foods rich in vitamin B6 and B12 can help in easing asthma.

- The Ginkgo biloba herb is also effective in treating asthma attacks, as well as reducing the frequency of these attacks owing to its ginkgolide B content.

- Reducing the amount of salt intake and taking 2000 mg of Vitamin C an hour before exercising can help in relieving exercise-induced asthma.

- Add 2 teaspoons of fenugreek seeds to a glass of water and boil it till only half the solution remains. Drinking this solution once a day can help in reducing the frequency of attacks.

- As a preventive therapy, you can add some Bishop's weed to boiling water and inhale the fumes emitted from the solution every night before sleeping.

- Inhaling the smell of honey, or adding 2 spoons of honey to a glass of milk and drinking it can help in alleviating asthma symptoms.

- Crush a piece of turmeric into fine powder, add some honey to it (1 part turmeric powder and 2 parts honey) and eat it. This will help in curing asthma and related breathing problems.

More Natural Cures for Asthma..

Vegetables and Fruits:

As per the different studies and researches, the intake of fruits and vegetables minimize the risk of asthma in adults as well as children. Garlic proves to be an excellent medicine when consumed after boiling with milk. Ginger tea along with garlic is also used in the treatment of asthma. Turmeric powder mixed with milk is an effective medicine to treat asthma. Consumption of carrots and tomatoes, along with leafy vegetables, is helpful to keep asthma at bay.

Buteyko:

It is a breathing technique, developed by Konstantin Pavlovich Buteyko of Russia. The patient who uses this method for the treatment of asthma, follows shallow breathing exercises. The objective or purpose behind using this technique is the generation of carbon dioxide. CO_2 helps dilate the smooth muscles present in the respiratory system.

Butterbur:

It is a type of shrub, found in Asia, Europe and North America. Petasin and isopetasin, the constituents found in this plant, treat asthma by reducing the spasms in smooth muscles of the lungs. The treatment also reduces the inflammatory effects of asthma.

Omega Fatty Acids:

These fatty acids play an important role in the reduction of arachidonic acid. The arachidonic acid is a fat that is responsible for the inflammatory effect of asthma. Eicosapentaenoic acid (EPA) and docosahexaenoic acid (DHA) are the important omega-3 fatty acids that are used for the treatment. These are available in the form of capsules in drug stores.

Bromelain:

It is a protease enzyme, which is extracted from pineapples. Bromelain is known for its anti-inflammatory properties and thus, is used for the treatment of asthma.

Boswellia:

A herb that is used in Ayurvedic medicines. Boswellia is known to have an inhibitory effect on leukotrienes. The leukotriene is a harmful compound. It is one of the factors causing asthma.

The natural treatments used for asthma are mostly preventive in nature. According to some physicians, the natural cures for asthma are slow in their action. Thus, the natural cures should be used in tandem, with the conventional medicines discussed herein that are available for treating asthma.

Does Chlorine in Water Cause Asthma Attacks

Lastly, let's look at a commonly missed cause of asthma that is prevelant in a lot of today's homes, chlorine. Recent some studies have revealed convincing results that point out chlorine as a potential asthma trigger. We all know that swimming is an excellent cardio workout, but when done in the chlorinated pools daily, it may eventually harm the lung tissue, leading to asthma. So, asthma sufferers are likely to experience worsening of their symptoms when swimming in the chlorinated water. Now, why chlorine and asthma do not go well together, is discussed below:

Chlorinated Water and Asthma

Those who are under the impression that chlorinated water cannot aggravate or cause asthma symptoms should first consider this data: The team manager of swimming team representing the United States in 2000 Olympics made an announcement that made their rival teams leap with joy. He announced that 25% of the team is not completely fit as some of the swimmers are diagnosed with asthma. Although the swimmers were not at all suffering from severe asthma, however it pointed out a link between chlorine and asthma risk.

Basically, chlorine is a disinfectant, and hence, is added in swimming pools to destroy the harmful microbes. However, it is observed that while swimming, chlorine combines with the swimmers' sweat, saliva, hair follicles, skin cells, cosmetics and even urine to release a number of chemical compounds known as Trihalomethanes (THMs). THMs that are also formed when chlorine reacts with water, are the ones that can induce and worsen the asthma.

Now, the question arises, if the swimmer is not drinking the pool water, how do these chemicals gain access to the lungs? The answer is quite simple - although these chemicals are in solid or liquid state, upon reaching the surface of the water, they turn volatile. Once they become volatile, they readily combine with air, which is inhaled frequently while swimming. Thus, the surrounding air acts as a medium of transportation for the THMs to the lungs. So, one can say that vapors of chlorinated water, when inhaled regularly can cause asthma.

A frequent exposure to THMs, results in inflammation of the lining of the respiratory tract, eventually triggering asthma symptoms. This happens because these water disinfectants are notorious for irritating the respiratory tract. Hence, their inhalation triggers an inflammatory response, resulting in narrowing of airways and subsequently causing asthma. No wonder, an increasing number of lifeguards and swim coaches complain about asthma symptoms. Their jobs demand staying near or inside the swimming pool for longer amounts of time. This in turn, prolongs their exposure to environment high in THMs, thereby making them susceptible to asthma.

In one study, it was observed that changing the environment of lifeguards and swimming coaches helped to improve their asthma considerably. In fact, asthma symptoms vanished after a certain period of time. This again proved that staying in an environment high in THMs contributes to the development of asthma.

Swimming pool environment does harm the lungs was also evident from another study. In the study, around 200 subjects who were school going kids in the age group of 8-10, had been asked to sit near the swimming pool for just over 15 minutes everyday. The study was continued for a specific duration of time and then results specifying the health of their lungs were examined carefully. It was observed that the lung tissues showed deterioration in varying degrees depending upon how long they stayed near the swimming pool. The study concluded that environment laden with THMs contributes to lung tissue damage and triggers asthma.

In another study, it was found that the risk of asthma due to chlorinated swimming pools is higher in people who are sensitive to allergies. The study in which approximately 850 children in the age group of 13-18 participated was conducted under the supervision of Belgian scientists. The result showed that children who are susceptible to allergies and swimming in chlorinated water have a higher chance of contracting asthma. Further the study concluded that chances of occurrence of asthma increase by almost 15 times in allergy sensitive children who are spending over 1000 hours in chlorinated water in their lifetime.

Considering the health hazards of swimming in chlorinated pools, is there any other way to clean the pool water? The research conducted by Belgian scientists also had a good news in store for competitive swimmers. The scientists after analyzing the condition of all the participants concluded that cleaning pools with copper or silver based disinfectants does not have any negative impact on health. To be more specific, healthy individuals taking a dip in swimming pools that contain silver/copper based disinfectants are unlikely to suffer from respiratory disorders. Using disinfectants that are a combination of chlorine and copper/silver ions is also a good option. This method effectively lowers the concentration of chlorine in pools, which helps to reduce the risk of asthma.

Chlorine Side Effects

Chlorine alone is not stable and hence, is always found in its compound form, the most common being sodium chloride and sodium hypochlorite. The one that is added to a swimming pool is usually sodium hypochlorite. Although chlorine added in water kills bacteria and protects us from water-borne illnesses, its vapors are said to be toxic. Chlorine gas is poisonous and when inhaled can trigger respiratory damage. Inhalation of chlorine gas for long periods of time can even cause death. Too much chlorine in pool water can also irritate the eyes and nose. Eyes becoming red is one of the most common side effects of swimming in chlorinated water. Small studies also suggest that swimming in the chlorinated pools and even taking a bath in chlorinated water daily increases the risk of various types of cancer.

Keep in mind that there are no extensive studies that confirm chlorinated pools as a major contributor to asthma attack. Yet, one should be extra careful when it comes to swimming in pools. Swimmers are advised to take a shower before entering the swimming pool. A proper shower bath will remove most of the dead skin cells that combine with chlorine to form harmful chemical compounds. Adding freshwater to swimming pools on a regular basis and urinating in the toilet (and not in the pool) can go a long way in minimizing exposure to THMs. Toddlers and small children have the habit of urinating in pools. So, as parents, you should not hesitate to take your children as often as possible to the toilet room.

On the whole, swimming everyday is no doubt a healthy way to keep the body in a good shape. However, make sure you choose the right swimming pool so as to prevent this outdoor activity from becoming harmful to your existing asthma condition.

Conclusion

Now you are familiar with the various types of asthma, whom they affect and common symptoms and cures. One important point to remember is that these home remedies should not be used as a substitute for prescribed medications. In cases where a person is suffering from severe asthma and undergoing asthma attack treatment, he should stick to asthma inhalers or asthma nebulizers recommended by the doctors.

Other than resorting to these common remedies, altering your way of life can also help in ensuring that you don't suffer from asthma attacks. Like we discussed, it is imperative that you identify the asthma triggers, like the foods, smells, allergens etc. which aggravate the respiratory ailment in your case, and try to avoid them at all costs. Asthma attacks can be very discomforting indeed, but with some simple precautionary measures on your behalf, you can make sure that asthma is kept at bay and you can once again BREATH EASY!